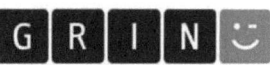

Marc Bonenberger

Famines. Understanding the Causes of Hunger and Disease in Sub-Saharan Africa

GRIN Publishing

Bibliographic information published by the German National Library:

The German National Library lists this publication in the National Bibliography; detailed bibliographic data are available on the Internet at http://dnb.dnb.de .

Imprint:

Copyright © 2009 GRIN Verlag GmbH
Print and binding: Books on Demand GmbH, Norderstedt Germany
ISBN: 978-3-656-89285-4

This book at GRIN:

http://www.grin.com/en/e-book/289018/famines-understanding-the-causes-of-hunger-and-disease-in-sub-saharan

GRIN - Your knowledge has value

Since its foundation in 1998, GRIN has specialized in publishing academic texts by students, college teachers and other academics as e-book and printed book. The website www.grin.com is an ideal platform for presenting term papers, final papers, scientific essays, dissertations and specialist books.

Visit us on the internet:

http://www.grin.com/

http://www.facebook.com/grincom

http://www.twitter.com/grin_com

Centre for African Studies Basel
University of Basel
Spring Term 2009

FAMINES

Understanding the Causes of Hunger and Disease in Sub-Saharan Africa

Research paper for the course 'Current Ecological and Health Issues'

Marc Bonenberger

M. A. African Studies

Basel, 20. May 2009

CONTENTS

List of Abbreviations.. ii

List of Figures iii

1. Introduction 1

2. Theorising Famine 4

   2.1. Natural Causes 4

   2.2. Panarchy, or Coupled Human-Ecological Systems 6

   2.3. Testing the Limits of Panarchy.. 10

3. Health Impacts 13

   3.1. Protein-Energy Malnutrition (PEM) 14

   3.2. Micronutrient Deficiencies... 17

   3.3. Infectious Diseases.. 19

4. Halving Extreme Poverty and Hunger in Africa? 22

   4.1. Strategies and Actions... 23

   4.2. Major Threats.. 24

      4.2.1. Food Price Crisis 24

      4.2.2. Climate Change 26

   4.3. Energy Crisis 28

5. Conclusions 30

6. Bibliography 32

List of Abbreviations

ARI   Acute Respiratory Infection

ASAL   Arid and Semi-Arid Land

ASPO   Association for the Study of Peak Oil and Gas

BMI   Body Mass Index

CDCP   Centre for Disease Control and Prevention

ENSO   El Niño Southern Oscillation

FAD   Food Availability Decline

FAO   Food and Agriculture Organisation

GHG   Greenhouse Gas

GHI   Global Hunger Index

HAZ   Height-for-Age Z-score

IFPRI   International Food Policy Research Institute

IPCC   Intergovernmental Panel on Climate Change

IRS   Indoor Residual Spraying

MDGs   Millennium Development Goals

MUAC   Mid Upper Arm Circumference

NCHS   US National Centre for Health Statistics

NCPB   National Cereals and Produce Board of the Kenyan Government

NGO   Non-Governmental Organisation

PEM   Protein-Energy Malnutrition

SCHR   Steering Committee for Humanitarian Response

SD   Standard Deviation

URR   Ultimate Recoverable Resources

UN   United Nations

UNICEF   United Nations Children's Fund

UNDP   United Nations Development Programme

WFP   World Food Programme

WHO   World Health Organisation

WHZ   Weight-for-Height Z-score

List of Figures

1. A Model of Famine Sequences 2

2.1. Adaptive Cycle 7

2.2. Panarchy 8

3.1. The 'Starvation Model' in contrast to the 'Health Crisis Model' 13

3.2. Causes of deaths among children under 5 years of age 19

4.1. The FAO Price Index 25

4.2. Atmospheric concentrations of CO_2 in pre-industrial times and in recent years 27

4.3. Hubbert's Peak 28

1. Introduction

In March 2006, after having visited a hospital in Garissa, a city in the North Eastern Province of Kenya, journalist Anna Badkhen reported in the San Francisco Chronicle: *'The baby was hungry. Habiba Mohammed pulled down the top of her dress and offered her emaciated child a breast that had not had milk for months. Her daughter, Hadiwa, is a casualty of a sustained, four-year drought that is threatening the lives of 17 million people across East Africa. Her ankles are no thicker than an adult's thumb; wrinkled skin hangs loosely around her thighs and angular pelvic bones. She is 9 months old and weighs 8 pounds, just over a pound more than her birth weight. Tuberculosis, malaria and pneumonia are eating away at her tiny body'* (Badkhen 2006).

Two years later, in July 2008, journalist Mark Lang visited the highland village Gale Wargo in southern Ethiopia. When asking Matheus, father of a three year old boy who is showing symptoms of acute wasting, how he and his family experienced the drought, he explained: *'The rain stopped back in September and we've had hardly any rain since then, so we lost our crops. We used to have an ox and two cows but they died because of the drought. There was some rain in April so we planted maize, but the yield will be low. The rainfall has not been good. Although it may look green and that there's a lot of growth, it's not uniform. We're not sure whether we will get a good harvest for the coming season. It's only God that knows what will happen'.* Grandmother Malaka adds: *'Look at us. This is the outcome of the food shortage. We are not in a position to give the children enough to eat'* (Lang 2008).

Despite the fact that there is currently enough food in the world for all, the poorest billion of the world's population is suffering from starvation and hunger-related diseases. Even though the last two decades saw a reduction in famines in other parts of the world, on the African continent it is still a sad reality (Devereux 2000). Scenes like the ones quoted above are recurring over and over again not only in Eastern Africa, but also in many other regions of sub-Saharan Africa.

There are numerous factors causing a famine, most importantly natural disasters, policy failures, conflicts and wars, production and market failures. In most cases it is not a single factor triggering a famine, but it is rather the result of interlocking processes. According to Dyson and ó Gráda (2002) famine sequences usually involve the following components (Fig. 1): At first, there are external events triggering a famine. These events usually are natural

1

calamities, such as drought, flood, frost, or a cold summer, and/or socio-political events, such as warfare, political isolation, policy-induced structural shifts, or economic disruption. In turn, these triggers cause hunger and starvation, either through food availability decline (FAD) or through a mismatch between food supply and effective demand in the population. The next components of the famine sequence are socio-economic effects, such as rise in food prices, migration of people, and social disruption. In turn, these processes again cause hunger and starvation and spread disease. Finally, among other demographic effects, such as decreased fertility, the most important is the rise in deaths. Hence, a famine can then be defined as *"a widespread and extreme hunger that results for individuals in a drastic loss of body weight and an increase in morbidity, and, at the community level, [...] in a rise in the death rate and massive social dysfunction and dislocation"* (Braun et al. 1998: 6).

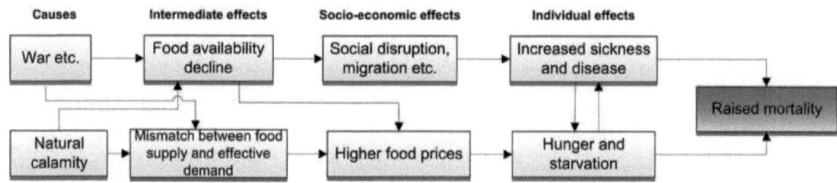

Figure 1: A Model of Famine Sequences (After Dyson and ó Gráda 2002: 13)

As indicated above, excess mortality is the characteristic feature of most famines. However, it is difficult to measure and calculations of famine attributable deaths in most cases are only educated guesses. This is due to a number of reasons: First, governments or non-governmental organisations (NGOs) often conceal or exaggerate food crises for political reasons or to mobilise humanitarian support. Second, in developing countries basic statistics are often unreliable or unavailable, and therefore excess mortality rates during famines cannot be compared with "normal" mortality rates. Third, famine mortality is often monitored in refugee camps, where people arrive already severely weakened and are exposed to an increased risk of infectious diseases. Under such conditions, the death rate is often elevated compared to other conditions, and hence care is needed to interpret these.

However, on the basis of available data, Devereux (2000) estimated that in the 20th century between 70 and 80 million people died in famines worldwide. For the African region alone, he estimated around 4 million famine deaths in the same period. Here, the most dramatic events occurred in Ethiopia of the 1950s and the 1970s where in total up to

800,000 people lost their lives after extended droughts. An additional 1 million were killed in the 1980s where conflicts worsened the already fatal drought situation. These numbers appear extraordinarily high, but compared to other parts of the world – for instance China, where more than 30 million (!) people lost their lives between 1958 and 1962 in a famine induced by policy failure (ibid.) – in fact this is relatively low.

The intention of this paper is threefold: The first chapter is an attempt to explain the causes of famines. Following the model of famine sequences of Dyson and ó Gráda (2002) the natural as well as socio-political causes of famines are included. However, differing from most other authors, who explained the causes of famines exclusively from the perspective of their own academic disciplines, a recent interdisciplinary model is used in this paper. The model, which was introduced by Gunderson and Holling in 2002, is called the *Panarchy* framework. It derives from an interdisciplinary approach that seeks to explain the mechanisms of creative destruction and renewal through which all ecological and human systems are assumed to cycle. That this model is useful also in the context of famine causation was demonstrated by Fraser (2003), who applied the framework to explain the causes of the Irish Potato Famine in the mid-19th century. In the present paper, the model of Gunderson and Holling (2002) is outlined at first and then tested on two cases of severe food shortages after prolonged droughts in Ethiopia and Kenya on the African continent in 1984-85. The ambition is also to prove the universal validity of the model when applied to famines.

Whatever the reasons for famines may be, the outcome is most likely the same: starvation and hunger-related diseases for the most vulnerable part of the population. The death rate increases due to severe malnutrition, usually defined as protein-energy malnutrition (PEM) and micronutrient deficiency. The immune system of affected persons becomes weakened and this predisposes them to infectious diseases. Thus, a vicious cycle emerges, because infection reduces appetite, decreases food intake and depletes the body of micronutrients. In the second chapter, the relationship between hunger, undernutrition and both communicable and non-communicable diseases will be explored. This includes the question, how undernutrition is measured and which relief practices in emergency situations are usually being applied.

At the Millennium Summit in the year 2000, leaders of 189 nation states assembled at the United Nations (UN) headquarters in New York City to ratify the UN Millennium Declaration. The declaration includes eight development goals, above all the overarching goal of halving extreme poverty and hunger by the year 2015. As this is a very challenging goal particularly for Africa, the only continent where poverty and hunger currently is increasing, in the third chapter, the strategies needed to meet the extreme poverty and hunger development goal are being explored. As there are a number of threats endangering the achievement of this goal, in a second part of this chapter the main threats are identified to deliberate about whether or not this goal may be achieved in Africa.

The overall research question is then how famines are caused, what effects they have on human health, and how the chances are to reduce poverty and hunger in Africa?

2. Theorising Famine

2.1. Natural Causes

All ecosystems are exposed to gradual changes in climate, nutrient loading, habitat fragmentation or biotic exploitation. Organisms have evolved mechanisms to absorb these changes and therefore ecosystems do not change easily to different states. However, stochastic events like fire, drought, disease epidemics, or biological invasion can cause sudden drastic switches to alternate states, which might have serious consequences on human well-being. Whether such switches occur depends on the resilience and the vulnerability of the ecosystem (Scheffer et al. 2001; Folke et al. 2002).

To challenge earlier static views that described nature in a steady state or near-equilibrium, Holling (1973) introduced the concept of resilience in ecological systems. In his classic paper, published in the *Annual Review of Ecology and Systematics*, he elaborated on the relationship between resilience and stability and described models of change in the structure and function of ecosystems. Today, Holling's notion of resilience is an important concept for a deeper understanding, management, and governing integrated systems of people and nature (Walker et al. 2006a), including diseases such as malaria (Obrist et al. 2007).

Holling did not deny that ecosystems can stabilise near an equilibrium steady state. After disturbances these systems are perceived to return rapidly to the original state. For this mechanism, later in his career, he shaped the term *engineering resilience*. But he strongly insisted that emphasis on this definition of resilience *"reinforces the dangerous myth that the variability of natural systems can be effectively controlled, that the consequences are predictable, and that sustained maximum production is an attainable and sustainable goal"*

4

(Gunderson and Holling 2002: 28). Holling suggested the term *ecosystem resilience* for systems far from any equilibrium steady state. Ecosystem resilience is measured in terms of the magnitude of disturbance or shock an ecological system can absorb before it changes to *another* state, where it subsequently stabilises (Holling 1973). In this case it might be difficult to return a system to the initial stability domain it has left.

A large body of evidence exists for such shifts to alternative stable states. For instance, Scheffer et al. (2001) analysed catastrophic shifts in lake, coral reef, desert, ocean and woodland ecosystems and described such shifts after a stochastic event. In the case of woodlands the authors showed how these ecosystems may shift between dense wood cover and a grassy open landscape as alternative stable states. For Tanzania and Botswana this was explained by low herbivore numbers due to a combination of rinderpest epidemic and elephant hunting in a few decades following the 1890s, allowing the woodlands to regenerate. Once the woodlands were re-established, they could not be destabilised by grazers. However, as a result of the destruction of woodlands by human activity and the rapid increasing density of elephants in the region, these ecosystems are currently shifting back to the previous grassy open landscape state – with all the negative impacts on human residents.

The antonym of resilience is denoted vulnerability. When an ecosystem loses resilience, it becomes vulnerable to external shocks that previously could be absorbed. Vulnerability depends on the sensitivity of the system – i.e. the degree to which a system will respond to shocks such as droughts, storms or pest infestation – as well as the ability to adapt to the new condition. Therefore, vulnerability is a function of both the sensitivity and the resilience of the ecosystem (Kasperson and Kasperson 2001; Folke et al. 2002; Turner et al. 2003).

A good example how ecosystems lose resilience and then become vulnerable to external shocks was offered by Koppel et al. (1997). They described catastrophic vegetation shifts in the Sahel region of Africa. As the livestock numbers increased in millions from the 1950 onwards, perennial grasses were replaced irreversibly by annual vegetation, which was highly sensitive to disturbances. In years with relatively low precipitation rates, the herbaceous vegetation collapsed, leaving a vegetation consisting of a sparse cover of unpalatable annual herbs and unpalatable shrubs. As a result, these processes induced soil degradation as the sparse vegetation could not protect the soil against erosion and surface run-off of rain water, causing desertification and ultimately famine in various parts of the region.

2.2. Panarchy, or Coupled Human-Ecological Systems

When crop failure occurs after an environmental shock or other such disasters the affected region becomes vulnerable to famine. However, an interesting question arises, why in eastern Africa the extensive droughts of 1984-85 created one of the worst famines in Ethiopia's history, while neighbouring Kenya remained largely unaffected. To answer this question, it is not sufficient to simply concentrate on ecosystems. A better understanding of how human and natural systems interact is necessary to address questions on the factors influencing famines.

An interesting approach to integrated theory is followed by the *Resilience Alliance*, a multidisciplinary research organisation comprised of ecologists, economists, social scientists, and mathematicians. Their research results were published in 2002 in a book titled *Panarchy. Understanding Transformations in Human and Natural Systems*. Gunderson and Holling, two key persons behind this organisation and the editors of the book, wrote the theoretic background in their influential chapters about adaptive change and panarchies. Basing on a variety of concepts such as resilience, vulnerability, and adaptability, the authors develop a new systems theory, which they denote as the *Panarchy* framework. The name derives from Pan, the Greek god of nature, and notions of hierarchies. In their context, *hierarchy* is not used as a top-down sequence of authoritative control, but rather in the sense of semi-autonomous levels which communicate a small set of information or quantity of material to the next higher level. Panarchy is then defined as a "*hierarchical structure in which systems of nature and humans, as well as combined human-nature systems and social-ecological systems, are interlinked in never-ending adaptive cycles of growth, accumulation, restructuring, and renewal*" (Holling 2001: 392).

Gunderson and Holling (2002) hold that all systems cycle through periods of resource accumulation and collapse (Fig. 2.1.). These processes are based on three key characteristics: (i) the resilience of the system, (ii) the connectedness of individuals, and (iii) the potential available for change in the system. Resilience is used in the ecosystem sense as the capacity to absorb change without shifting to an altered state with different properties. Thus, it determines how vulnerable the system is to unexpected disturbances. Ecosystem resilience has already been discussed and exemplified earlier. Human systems are resilient when they are able to cope with change, i.e. when institutions and networks exist *'that learn and store knowledge and experience, create flexibility in problem solving and balance power among interest groups'* (Folke et al. 2002: 17). For example, when a region faces a crisis after an extensive period of drought, the situation is usually mitigated by the importation of resources from the state. Thus, the system is resilient and the afflicted region persists. But when many regions within the country encounter the same difficulties and have to be subsidised simultaneously, the poorest states will probably not be able to procure the needed resources and lose resilience. If the international community fails for any reason, such as civil war that prevents relief organisations to enter a region, to provide food aid and other services the crisis may then turn into a famine (Carpenter et al. 2001).

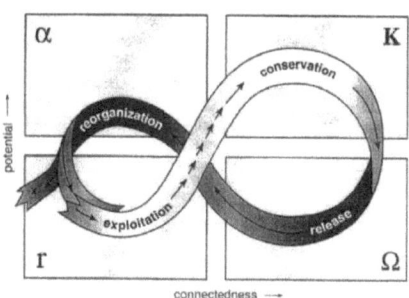

Figure 2.1. Adaptive Cycle
(Source: Gunderson and Holling 2002: 34)

Connectedness describes the degree of connectivity among the variables in the system. In a low connected system, all the variables exist, but are only loosely connected to one another. When the system is highly connected, the variables are tightly interconnected (Ostrom 2004). Vulnerabilities may arise when strong couplings of variables exist, since failure in one component has then greater impact upon other components than when variables are not tightly linked (Young et al. 2006). Applied to ecosystems, connectedness can be seen as the density of all animal, plant and human individuals living together within one system. The more crowded they live the more vulnerable they are to external forces. For instance, connectivity is higher in a dense forest ecosystem than in a loosely stocked plantation. In densely populated areas individuals are more vulnerable, because disasters such as fires or infectious diseases will spread faster than they would in loosely populated systems (Fraser 2003). Connectedness in human systems describes the connectivity of the different parts of human society in the social, cultural, political and economic sphere. On the one hand, the existence of many interconnections may enhance the resilience of the whole system by diluting and distributing the impact of strong changes in individual elements upon other elements of the system. On the other hand, interdependencies – such as of flows of

7

trade, information and people – between these parts arise as connectedness increases. When the system gets overconnected, disturbances may spread rapidly across the different parts of society (Young et al. 2006).

Potential for change determines the range of possible future options. In an ecosystem it refers to the accumulated resources in biomass that Gunderson and Holling (2002) loosely define as the wealth available in the system. Wealth can be measured in terms of the foliage that would provide food for an opportunistic pest, or biomass that could fuel a fire. A forest ecosystem can be regarded as a wealthy system, as it often has a rich foliage and a high biomass. According to this concept the system has a high potential for change and therefore is more susceptible to disturbances than is a non-wealthy system (Holling 2001, Gunderson and Holling 2002, Fraser 2003). In human systems, potential could be represented by the character of the accumulated networks of relationship – e.g. friendship, mutual respect, and trust among people and institutions of governance – as well as by the accumulated usable knowledge, inventions, and skills that are available and accessible. Gunderson and Holling (2002) claim, as potential increases social systems get increasingly rigid in its control. In some cases, rigid systems may face certain difficulties in responding adequately to extreme events.

According to the authors of *Panarchy*, all systems recover after a disturbance by accumulating wealth. When the potential and thus the wealth builds up, connectivity also increases. Hence, the resilience in the system decreases. As time passes by, the point is reached when the potential for change is high, connectivity is high, and resilience is low. The system becomes *"an accident waiting to happen"* (Holling 2001: 396). It is then possible that an external event may trigger a total collapse of the whole system. What then follows is a quick release of the accumulated wealth, which causes the system to revert to a less organized state. When this happens, it enters a new phase of reorganization that leads again to wealth accumulation, increased connectivity and reduced diversity (Gunderson and Holling 2002, Fraser et al. 2005).

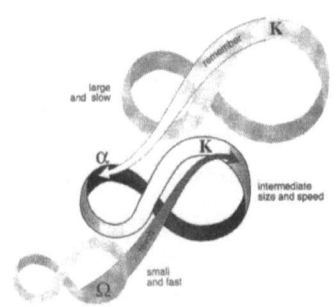

Figure 2.2. Panarchy
(Source: Gunderson and Holling 2002: 75)

The *Panarchy* framework holds that all ecological and human systems represent such

8

adaptive cycles that are nested one within each other across spatial scales, whereas the structure of these cycles is arranged hierarchical (Holling 2001, Fig. 2.2.). When one level in the panarchy experiences a disturbance and collapse, that collapse can cascade up to the next larger level by triggering a crisis. This may be particularly true if that level has also accumulated vulnerabilities and rigidities. This cascading effect Gunderson and Holling (2002) termed as a *revolt* connection. When many levels facing vulnerabilities and rigidities at the same time a revolt connection from the lowest to the highest level may lead to an entire collapse of the whole panarchy. On the other hand, upper levels in the panarchy may mitigate drastic situations faced by lower levels as they can draw on their potential that has been accumulated and stored previously: *"It is as if this connection draws upon the accumulated wisdom and experiences of maturity"* (ibid.: 76). For this reason, the authors termed this mitigating effect as a *remember* connection.

A food system, which is a human-ecological system, may be regarded as a panarchy. A food system is defined as *"a set of activities and outcomes ranging from production through to consumption, which involve both human and environmental dimensions"* (Ericksen 2008: 3). These systems can be regarded as a nested set of systems comprising of culture, politics, societies, economics, and ecosystems. All these systems are intertwined in a hierarchical order to one large system, whereas the upper levels, such as politics, protect the lower levels, such as ecosystems. Hence, they form a panarchy. Following Gunderson and Holling (2002), after a crisis occurred at one level of the food-system-panarchy it can be either mitigated by higher levels or spread across them. In the first case, higher levels, basing on their knowledge of former similar crises, would find solutions to mitigate the situation. In case that their mitigating attempts fail or if no solutions are at hand, the crisis worsens or may emerge into a famine. A famine would then represent a collapsing panarchy when all the levels of the systems fail by degrees. A scenario such as follows is conceivable: An external trigger, e.g. a drought or a flood, causing one level such as the agro-ecosystem to fail, resulting in a revolt connection which affects the next higher level such as the social system, which may subsequently cause hunger-related social disruption. In turn, social disruption may then be the trigger that causes the political system, as a higher level in the panarchy, to fail. As the political system breaks down as well, the situation may escalate into civil war, holding relief organisations off from entering the affected area. Eventually, while the whole panarchy collapses the emerging famine in the region worsens.

2.3. Testing the Limits of Panarchy

As the Panarchy framework seems to be a powerful concept to explain why famine evolve in theory, in this section its usefulness is to be proved in practice by exemplifying it in the context of historic famine events in Ethiopia and Kenya of 1984-85. Both countries in eastern Africa faced extensive droughts over successive years and became vulnerable to famine. But while Ethiopia experienced one of its worst famines which cost hundreds of thousands of lives, neighbouring Kenya solved the crisis without evolving a famine. What follows is an attempt to explain this fact in the context of the Panarchy framework.

Prolonged droughts and famines is a recurrent threat in Ethiopia's population and famines being traced back to the 3rd century BC (Unruh 2001). The most drought-prone regions are the north-eastern highlands, the eastern plains bordering Somalia, and the south adjacent to Kenya. Due to El Niño Southern Oscillation (ENSO) events and the long-range effects of Western industrial pollution (Nowak 2002), Ethiopia faced a decline in rainfalls since the 1960s, resulting in two major famines in 1973-74 and 1984-85, which together caused over 600,000 deaths in the country (Fraser 2007). When in the 1980s the rains consecutively failed, the northern provinces were struck first by drought, but from there it gradually expanded into the central highlands, and then progressed into the western semi-arid belt. After the crops had failed, people most vulnerable to famine where those who had few economic opportunities outside of agriculture (ibid.). This was especially true in the northern provinces of Ethiopia, to where, in the 1970s, the authoritarian Marxist military regime, known as the *Derge* and headed by General Mengistu Haile Mariam, forcefully transported people in an attempt to set up Soviet style agricultural communes (von Braun et al. 1999). The Derge, after initially denying the food crisis, reacted with a hasty and unorganised distribution of stored grain. As the attempts of the government to provide relief failed, those provinces traditionally discontented with the central government accused the Derge of policy failures. As social restlessness increased regional militias emerged that started guerrilla warfare against the regime. As a result of combined severe food shortages and civil war, the food crisis turned into a famine (Comenetz and Caviedes 2002, Fraser 2007).

Also in Kenya drought is a potential hazard for agriculture in nearly all provinces of the country (Nyamwange 1995). Embracing the Rift Valley, the north-eastern and eastern provinces and the Coast Province, 80% of Kenya is classified as arid and semi-arid land

(ASAL). The ASALs are the regions usually most affected by drought. Agriculture generates almost all of the country's food requirements and 75% of the population earns its living from this activity (UNDP 2004). As much of the agriculture practised by the peasants is rain-fed, food production relies heavily on sufficient seasonal rainfall amounts (Speranza et al. 2008). Beginning in 1983 in northern and north-eastern Kenya, in 1984 almost the entire country was hit by drought, resulting in serious losses of cereal stocks: Compared to normal years, production of maize, the nation's principal staple food crop, declined by up to 50%, wheat and potato production, both major crops, were even up to 70% below normal (cf. Nyamwange 1995, von Braun et al. 1999). Worst affected were the provinces around Nairobi, the capital city of Kenya in the central highlands. The Kenyan government, then under presidency of Daniel arap Moi, established an interministry drought response committee and responded to the catastrophe in a timely and expeditious fashion. They began importing large amounts of maize and wheat to meet demands. The government's initial response was based on several factors, such as meteorological reports, accounts from the district administration and field staff of different NGOs, and the rapid increase in maize sales by the National Cereals and Produce Board (NCPB). Additionally, politicians could visualise the extent of the crisis as the most fatal drought was centred in and around Nairobi. The imported food was distributed through the normal commercial channels, and thereby keeping prices stable. Support to vulnerable households in the affected areas was also conducted. When in 1985 the long rains were about average, the drought emergency was considered over. Nevertheless, the government provided food aid during the recovery phase and until the next harvest (ibid.).

Following the Panarchy approach of Gunderson and Holling (2002), the Kenyan food system of the years 1984-85 can be regarded as a healthy system. When the agro-ecosystem collapsed after consecutive droughts, the social system as the next higher level in the panarchy lost resilience and became vulnerable to famine. A breakdown of the social system and a revolt connection to the economic system was prevented by the political system, as it provided adequate and timely relief in the form of food aid, and thus preventing hunger, starvation and disease across the country. Moreover, a remember connection between the political and the economic system was established as the food was mostly distributed through commercial channels. This prevented the prices of important cereals to explode, as it often happens in such situations. Hence, remember connections from the political system to the economic system to the social system had had stabilising effects to the whole panarchy.

The example of Ethiopia in the same period represents a collapsing panarchy. For similar reasons as in Kenya, the country's agro-ecosystem collapsed and established a revolt connection to the social system, which subsequently became vulnerable to famine. In this case, the political system as a larger level in the panarchy did not protect the lower levels, but rather worsened the situation by implementing specific policies. Not only had the government deracinated people from their own communities and transported them to distinct areas where they lost social ties. Furthermore, its delayed reaction to the food crisis and latter awkward attempts to provide relief also contributed to an aggravation of this crisis. These failed mitigating attempts caused further social unrest. This resulted in a revolt connection from the social system to the political system, which in turn lost resilience. Eventually, due to both the occurrence of civil war and the aggravation of the food crisis the whole panarchy collapsed into famine.

These findings show that the concept of nested cycles put forth by Gunderson and Holling (2002) has to be slightly modified when applied to famines. As written earlier in this paper, the authors hold that higher levels in the panarchy, by establishing a remember connection, are able to 'protect' lower levels in the system and thereby preventing them collapsing. However, the example of Ethiopia clearly demonstrates that higher levels are equally able to establish revolt connections with the lower levels.

More problems arise when turning towards the individual levels of the panarchy. Gunderson and Holling (2002) claim that high connectivity and wealth reduce resilience of a system. However, when applied to social systems, high connectivity often *increases* resilience, since well connected communities are often better able to adapt to unexpected problems. Moreover, wealth with respect to capital (be it financial, social or political capital) reduces the vulnerability of the person or the community that owns it (Fraser et al. 2005 and Fraser 2007). In the context of Ethiopia's famine, these issues explain why those people with weak social ties suffered the most. A similar objection can be raised regarding the political system in Kenya: Having well connected and collaborating political institutions had helped the country to provide relief in a timely manner, and thereby decreasing vulnerability to the whole food system. For this reasons, other authors working on famine and who faced the same problems when applying the Panarchy framework, tend to replace the concepts of potential and connectivity with the concept of *capital* (see for instance Abel et al. 2006; Walker et al. 2006b). Abel et al. (2006) broadly define capital as "*a stock with the potential to yield a flow of benefits*" (3). The authors prefer this concept, because, as they argue, it is better able to explain why human-ecological systems may collapse. Not only does capital capture both potential and connectedness in human-ecological systems, but it also includes the concept of *adaptive capacity*, which refers to the human ability to develop and adopt novel solutions when faced by a broad range of challenges (ibid.). Abel et al. (2006) therefore describe the dynamics of human-ecological systems in terms of social, human, natural, physical and financial capital. In this sense, the loss of capital can trigger a collapse of one system which then may cascade up or down to other systems in the panarchy.

Despite these objections the Panarchy framework is a promising approach to explain why famines evolve and it has proved useful in a number of studies (see for instance Berkes et al. 2002, Fraser 2003). However, at this stage of development it is a good advice not to take the framework too literally and to rather take it as what it actually is: a metaphor.

3. Health Impacts

As indicated in the introductory part, excess mortality is the characteristic feature in most famines. However, in most cases victims are not simply starving to death, as it is often stated in the media. Even though hunger may be the underlying cause of death, people are more often than not dying from infectious diseases. To explain famine mortality most authors adopt the 'starvation model'. This model stresses that lack of food consumption is the trigger of excess mortality, as the body of malnourished people becomes increasingly susceptible to infectious diseases. Therefore, this

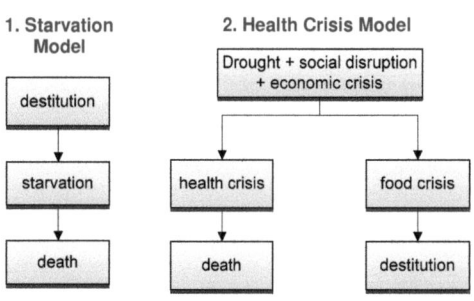

Figure 3.1. The 'Starvation Model' in contrast to the 'Health Crisis Model' (After de Waal 2005 [1989]: 187, 189)

model suggests that diseases as a result of malnutrition are the proximate causes of death (Fig. 3.1). Alex de Waal (2005 [1989]), the author of 'Famine that kills. Darfur, Sudan', has a somewhat different hypothesis. When he conducted research for his PhD in Darfur during the famine of 1984-85 in Sudan he could not affirm the link between destitution and mortality. He observed that mortality did not increase due to increased susceptibility to infections, but rather to increased *exposure* to potentially fatal diseases. As many people migrated out of the most afflicted rural areas and concentrated in the cities, the public health environment became degraded. Not only did the quality and the quantity of water decline, but also did migrants bring diseases to their hosts. In Darfur both aspects accelerated the rates of transmission of infectious diseases, which resulted, in de Waal's words, in a 'health crisis' and increased mortality. Therefore, he suggests a 'Health Crisis Model' (Fig. 3.1) instead of the 'Starvation Model', at least for the situation in Darfur. This model does not deny that famine causes destitution and death, but it holds that famine causes death in parallel to destitution, and not because of it.

However, de Waal (2005 [1989]) admitted the possibility that his sample had not been large enough to draw this conclusion, and if it had, some of the variances in death rates could probably have been explained by measurements of poverty and malnutrition. Another objection is that as in Darfur mortality did rise due to increased exposure to infectious diseases it is possible that rather malnourished people died, who were more susceptible to infections, than those better nourished. Yet, de Waal's 'Health Crisis Model' cannot be dismissed completely, as its argumentation is logical and comprehensible. However, further research is needed to prove its validity.

This chapter follows more the 'traditional' supposition of the starvation model, which holds that increased mortality occurs due to both severe malnutrition and increased susceptibility to infectious diseases. PEM, micronutrient deficiencies and infectious diseases are examined and contrasted with each other. This includes the question, how malnutrition is measured and which relief practices in emergency situations are usually applied by health workers in the field.

3.1. Protein-Energy Malnutrition (PEM)

Since access to food is limited during famines affected persons often suffer from PEM. PEM arises when the diet is quantitatively or qualitatively inadequate – i.e. when it is unbalanced and deficient in particular nutrients (Waterlow 1997). While it is estimated that about 760 million people in various parts of the developing world are currently chronically malnourished and have milder forms of PEM, approximately 85 million people are acutely malnourished and face severe PEM (UN Millennium Project 2005). According to the *Guidelines for care at the first-referral level in developing countries* of the World Health Organisation (WHO 2000), severe PEM occurs when kwashiorkor, marasmus or clinical signs of severe malnutrition are visible. Kwashiorkor mainly occurs in persons with insufficient protein consumption. The symptoms are serious weight loss accompanied by a swollen abdomen, the presence of oedema, reddish discolouration of the hair, and depigmented skin. Marasmus arises when energy intakes are extremely low. Here the symptoms are extensive tissue and muscle wasting (Waterlow 1997). Under normal conditions both marasmus and kwashiorkor are extremely rare, but they are likely to occur in emergency situations, such as famine and war. In the case diseased persons cannot be treated immediately, they are at high risk of dying from severe malnutrition (UNICEF 1998: 14).

While it is relatively easy to identify persons with severe PEM, the signs and symptoms of milder forms are not obvious to untrained observers and are difficult to standardise. For this reason, clinical diagnoses are seldom used in the field. Because PEM is associated with growth failure or retardation, it is more effective to use anthropometric criteria instead. Therefore, health workers usually assess the nutritional status of children below the age of 5 years as a proxy for the nutritional status of the whole community (Salama et al. 2001, De Onis and Blössner 2003). When using anthropometric criteria the size and growth of the children in the community are measured with reference to children in a well-nourished population – for instance, by using US National Centre for Health Statistics (NCHS)/WHO reference values (Berkley et al. 2005). According to WHO (1995) recommendations, the anthropometric indices should hereby being expressed in terms of Z-scores[1] (or standard deviation scores). By comparing the size, and thus the weight for the height, the relative thinness of a child is measured. The WHO (2000) defines a weight-for-height Z-score (WHZ) below -2 standard deviation (SD) as wasting and a WHZ below -3 SD as severe wasting. By comparing the growth of a child, and thus the height for the age, the relative shortness is measured. A height-for-age Z-score (HAZ) below -2 SD the WHO defines as stunting. Unless stunted children are not severely wasted or have a serious illness they do not require hospital admission. Severely wasted children, however, are extremely malnourished and are indicators of high PEM prevalence in the community (CDCP 1992). Therefore, measuring

---

[1]A Z-score is *'the deviation of the value for an individual from the median value of the reference population, divided by the standard deviation for the reference population'* (WHO 1995: 7).

WHZ Z-scores is a good predictor of subsequent mortality in community-based studies. However, Berkley et al. (2005) criticise WHO recommendations of using WHZ Z-scores to measure severe malnutrition in sub-Saharan Africa, because, basing on their experience with Kenyan food crises, (i) height is difficult to measure accurately in ill or distressed children, and (ii), perhaps more important, the measurement of weight depends on the presence of properly calibrated functioning scales, which are often not available. Therefore, Berkley et al. propose to use mid upper arm circumference (MUAC) instead, because it is *'a simple, low cost, objective method of assessing nutritional status'* (592).

The practice of including children as the only demographic group in nutrition surveys is contested as well. For instance, Salama et al. (2001), who had worked in Ethiopia during the famine of 1998-2000, note that by the time NGOs began operating, in some provinces the most severely wasted children had already died. Finding low prevalence of wasting often led to the erroneous conclusion that the nutritional status of the population was stable or improving. Therefore, Salama et al. (2001) stress the importance of including adults and older persons in nutrition surveys as well to assessing mortality of a community during prolonged, severe famines. The authors identify the lack of consensus among international agencies on the most suitable anthropometric indicator and anthropometric cut-offs for defining adult undernutrition as a main reason that adults are regularly not included in these surveys. Salama et al. propose to use body mass index (BMI[2]) cut-offs in the field. However, for this measures they admit that in case that no healthy reference population of the same ethnicity is present, the lack of comparability between ethnic groups that results from variation in body shape may make it difficult to implicate. Woodruff and Duffield (2002), who regularly included measurement of BMI of adolescents in their nutrition surveys in various emergency situations in Africa and Asia, add that during severe famines where adolescents and adults are affected, many of the most severely malnourished cannot stand, making measurement of height impossible. However, both Salama et al. (2001) and Woodruff and Duffield (2002) conclude that until better methods can be developed and validated, health workers should use BMI to detect severe malnutrition also in other population subgroups than children. This would also *'challenge the assumption that only children younger than 5 years are at a higher risk for malnutrition and mortality'* (Salama et al. 2001: 570).

---

[2]BMI is *'a simple index of weight-for-height that is commonly used to classify underweight, overweight and obesity in adults. It is defined as the weight in kilograms divided by the square of the height in metres (kg/m^2)'* (WHO 2009: URL: http://www.who.int/bmi/index.jsp?introPage=intro_3.html [08.04.2009]).

3.2. Micronutrient Deficiencies

Although a lack of energy and protein is associated with increased risk of mortality due to starvation, in most famines it is not usually identified as a major cause of death. More important than adequacy in total food consumption is the *quality* of the food consumed. Much crisis-related mortality can therefore be ascribed to an unbalanced diet that is deficient in particular *micronutrients* (Webb and Thorne-Lyman 2005). UNICEF (1998) defines micronutrients as nutrients that are needed by the body only in minute amounts, but which are essential *'for the production of enzymes, hormones and other substances that are required to regulate biological processes leading to growth, activity, development and the functioning of the immune and reproductive systems'* (14). Micronutrients usually come from non-staple foods, such as animal products (e.g. meat, eggs, milk), vegetables and fruits, which the poorest population often cannot afford or which are simply not available during famines or other crises situations. Deficiencies in micronutrients can lead to serious health problems, including reduced resistance to infectious diseases, blindness, lethargy, reduced learning capacity, mental retardation and even death (UNICEF 1998, Ekweagwu et al. 2008). Therefore, the delivery of adequate food in terms of micronutrients is now recognised as a key aspect in relief operations during famines. However, micronutrient deficiencies occur not only in emergency situations, but are widespread also under normal conditions in the developing world and affect approximately 2 billion people, which is about one third of the world's population. Because people deficient in micronutrients do not necessarily feel hungry and are largely unaware of the deficiencies that they face this kind of malnutrition is often called "hidden hunger" (Webb and Thorne-Lyman 2005, WFP 2007).

The World Food Programme (WFP 2007) singled out vitamin A, iron, zinc, and folate as of particular importance for public health. Deficiencies in the first three micronutrients even rank among the top 10 leading causes of death through disease in developing countries (WHO 2002). Vitamin A is vital for the body, because it helps to regulate the immune system, growth, vision reproduction and cellular differentiation. Vitamin A deficiency accounts for several health problems. During pregnancy it increases the risk of maternal mortality and in infants and young children of dying from diarrhoea, measles, pneumonia, malaria and other diseases. It also increases the risk of blindness, respiratory diseases and chronic ear infection. Iron is an important micronutrient, because it helps to produce energy by carrying oxygen to red blood cells. Iron deficiency in pregnant women increases the risk of low birth weight and perinatal morbidity and mortality. In infants, young and older children it increases the risk of anaemia and acute respiratory infections and decreases their learning capacity. Zinc is essential for the body, because it plays a catalytic role in over 100 specific metabolic enzymes in human metabolism. It is found virtually in every tissue in the body and is particularly important for the correct functioning of the immune system, growth and development and the antioxidant system. As animal protein is the richest source of zinc, deficiency in this micronutrient is one of the most prevalent nutritional disorders during famines. Zinc deficiency is associated with difficulties during pregnancies and childbirth. It is also responsible for compromised immune responses and increases the risk of infectious diseases such as diarrhoea, pneumonia and malaria. Folate is a B-vitamin found in a variety of foods, but predominantly in dark green leafy vegetables. It is required for the synthesis of DNA, RNA, and protein, prime events for cellular replication and growth. Folate helps to reduce the risk of neurological defects in foetuses and for infants it is essential for the development of the neurological system. Deficiency of folate increases the risk of certain serious and common birth defects, which affects the brain and spinal cord. The most prominent are *spinal bifida*, which is a neural tube defect resulting in a wide range of physical disabilities, and *anencephaly*, another neural tube defect which may result in miscarriages, stillbirths or neonatal deaths. Beside these micronutrients, vitamins E, C, D, B_2 B_6, selenium, copper, and iodine are identified as important for public health as well (UNICEF 1998, Webb and Thorne-Lyman 2005, WFP 2007, Ekweagwu et al. 2008).

Because micronutrient deficiency does not manifest itself visually in a bloated belly or emaciated body it is difficult to assess. As assessments require qualified staff and training and often expensive high technology for biochemical tests, they have remained scarce during famines (Seal and Prudhon 2007). When implemented in nutrition surveys, health workers mainly use direct and indirect assessments to investigate micronutrient deficiencies. When using indirect assessments the nutrient intakes of the screened population is usually estimated on the basis of food frequency questionnaires, in which the survey subjects are asked whether they have consumed a specific food item or food group, typically within the last 24 hours or 7 days. By evaluating these questionnaires the diversity of the food consumed is measured to calculate the risk of deficiency in the population. Eventually, the prevalence and public health seriousness is extrapolated from the questionnaire data (Swindale and Bilinsky 2005). In direct assessments, health workers may use clinical signs and

18

biochemical testing as two main approaches to micronutrient deficiencies. Clinical signs are observed visually by surveyors or medical practitioners. Most health workers prefer this option as it is *'non-invasive, usually low cost, and is often the most logistically feasible option in remote areas'* (Seal and Prudhon 2007: 9). On the other hand, findings may be misleading as clinical signs are, with a few exceptions, often non-specific. For instance, goitre is considered as a specific clinical sign of iodine deficiency, but it is also possible that goitre results from iodine excess or some other disease processes. Biochemical tests have the advantage that nutritional deficiencies can be detected before the appearance of overt clinical signs. However, these tests are expensive, time consuming and cannot be applied on a large scale. Moreover, many nutrients are difficult to test accurately, because blood samples are not representative of the sites (such as enzyme systems, bone marrow, etc.) where the nutrient is stored or acts and therefore, the results obtained should not always be regarded as definitive. Nevertheless, biochemical tests can provide an invaluable additional tool in reaching conclusions (ibid.).

3.3. Infectious Diseases

As indicated in the previous sections, the main contribution of malnutrition to famine-related mortality is not through starvation, but rather through communicable diseases. This is due predominantly to undernourishment based on PEM as well as deficiency in micronutrients, since both types of malnutrition impair the immunity system and make the body more susceptible to infectious diseases (Schaible and Kaufmann 2007). In addition, this effect is aggravated in the worst affected regions as people often have to rely on contaminated 'famine food' and tend to migrate in search of assistance at crowded relief camps, where sanitation may be poor and clean water scarce, and

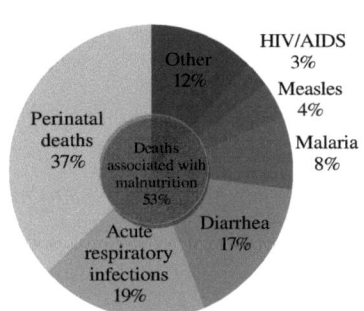

Figure 3.2. Causes of deaths among children under 5 years of age, 2000-2003, worldwide. 53 % of these cases are associated with malnutrition. (After Müller and Krawinkel 2005: 279)

hence infectious diseases are likely to spread out (von Braun et al. 1999, Dyson and Ó Gráda 2002). Moreover, infections can have serious impacts on nutritional status, because loss of appetite and impaired nutrient absorption are common concomitant features in affected persons (Ambrus and Ambrus 2004). Therefore, malnutrition and disease form a vicious cycle as the relationship between both is bidirectional and mutually reinforcing.

The most vulnerable of dying from infectious diseases are developing foetuses, children under to the age of 5 years and women before and during pregnancy and while they are breastfeeding (UNICEF 1998). As specified by Müller and Krawinkel (2005, Fig. 3.2.), the main causes of death from infectious diseases worldwide between 2000 and 2003 among children less than 5 years of age are acute respiratory infections (ARIs) (19%), diarrhoea (17%), malaria (8%), measles (4%), and HIV/AIDS (3%). 53 % of these cases were associated with malnutrition. As described by several authors these findings fit well also under famine conditions. For instance, de Waal (2005 [1989]) notes that in Sudan the leading causes of death among children were due to diarrhoeal diseases, measles, malaria or pneumonia. Salama et al. (2001) worked in neighboring Ethiopia some 20 years later during the famine at the end of the 20th century. They reported that among 4,032 people under observation in the Gode district, 293 deaths occurred during the period between December 1999 and July 2000, whereas 159 (54.3%) had been children younger than 5 years. 86% of these children died from measles, diarrhoea, malaria or respiratory tract infections in combination with severe wasting, and 30% deceased from one or more of these communicable diseases without showing signs of wasting. In contrast, for subjects over 60 years of age the respective percentages were 10% and 4%, whereas the total number of deaths in this age group was 24 (8.2%).

Diarrhoeal diseases and ARIs are both strongly associated with micronutrient deficiencies, as in undernourished children episodes of these diseases are likely to be more severe and of longer duration. In turn, diarrhoea and ARI are supposed to increase the risk for developing micronutrient deficiencies, particularly in vitamin A and zinc (WFP 2007). Cases of malaria tend to be more severe in persons suffering from PEM and micronutrient deficiencies, especially in children and pregnant women. Recent studies conducted in several African countries clearly demonstrated the relationship between malaria mortality and undernutrition, indicating that the risk of dying from this disease is 1.3 to 3.5 times higher in undernourished persons than in normally nourished people. Moreover, these studies state that some micronutrients such as vitamin A, zinc and iron have protective efficacies, although little is known of the mechanism leading to enhanced immunity to malaria infection

20

(Shankar 2000). Measles is one of the most contagious diseases known and large outbreaks could be observed during many famines, particularly in relief camps or in other situations where people had to live closely crowded. (Salama et al. 2001). Primarily malnourished children younger than 5 years are at high risk of death following an attack of measles, but the disease can also trigger acute PEM and worsen vitamin A deficiency (WHO 2005). HIV/AIDS is associated with undernutrition as well, as HIV-infected persons have increased energy demands. According to the WHO (2003) the energy needs among adults increase by 20-30%, among children even by 50-100%. However, access to sufficient quantity and quality of food is often limited during famines, which can then result in further nutritional decline.

To avoid illness and death from diarrhoea and infectious diseases transmitted by the faeco-oral route, the Sphere Project (2004), a programme of the Steering Committee for Humanitarian Response (SCHR), recommends in its handbook *Humanitarian Charter and Minimum Standards in Disaster Response* to set up water supply and sanitation programmes as soon as possible. These programmes should include the promotion of good hygiene practices, the provision of clean drinking water and the reduction of environmental health risks. In order to ensure that the entire affected population has access to clean water and adequate sanitation services, it is important to encourage women's participation in these programmes wherever possible. As measles has high potential for outbreak and mortality, measles immunisation should be implemented immediately. Prior to a mass vaccination campaign, an estimation of measles vaccination coverage of children aged 9 months to 15 years should be conducted. If vaccination coverage is estimated to be less than 90% or in the case the coverage is unknown, at least 95% of the children in this age group should receive measles vaccination (q.v. Salama et al. 2001). As outbreaks of other childhood diseases are less frequent and the health risks associated with them are lower, vaccination to these diseases is of lesser priority. Malaria incidence is likely to rise particularly in relief camps or in other situations were mass population movements are involved. Therefore, it should be ensured that appropriate chemoprophylaxis can be provided. As resistance to chloroquine and sulphadoxine-pyrimethamine is widespread and increasing, the provision of more efficacious anti-malarial drugs should be considered. In addition to medical treatment, vector control measures such as indoor residual spraying (IRS) and the distribution of insecticide-treated nets (ITNs) should be initiated. To decrease the risk of HIV/AIDS dissemination during disasters, the Sphere Project's handbook recommends that all people have access to free male condoms and the promotion of proper condom use, universal precautions to prevent iatrogenic/nosocomial transmission in emergency and health-care settings, and safe blood supply. Moreover, individuals should receive relevant information and education so that they can take steps to protect themselves against HIV transmission. All people already living with HIV/AIDS should be guaranteed basic health care.

4. Halving Extreme Poverty and Hunger in Africa?

At the 2000 UN Millennium Summit leaders from 189 nations gathered at the UN headquarters in New York City to ratify the UN Millennium Declaration. It included eight development goals, above all the overarching goal '*to halve, by the year 2015, the proportion of the world's people whose income is less than one dollar a day and the proportion of people who suffer from hunger [...]*' (5). It is estimated that more than 1 billion people in the world still face extreme poverty and that more than 800 million people go to bed hungry every day – among them 300 million are children (Millennium Project 2006). In Africa alone are living 200 million, or one fourth of the world's malnourished. Having a total population of almost 970 million people, this means that approximately every fifth African denizen is chronically or acutely malnourished (Millennium Project 2005). Moreover, sub-Saharan Africa is the only region in the world where poverty and hunger is increasing. 16 of the 20 countries with the highest Global Hunger Index (GHI[3]) scores are African countries, with the Democratic Republic of the Congo, Eritrea, Burundi, Niger and Sierra Leone at the bottom of the list (IFPRI 2008). In 2004, the share of the population living on less than US$ 1 a day was 41% and most of the people living on even less than US$ 0.50 a day – also called the ultra poor – were concentrated in this region (IFPRI 2008). In the face of these numbers, particularly for the African continent, the extreme poverty and hunger Millennium Development Goal (MDG) appears to be a very challenging, although desirable goal.

The purpose of this chapter is two-fold: In the first section the strategies needed to meet the extreme poverty and hunger MDG in sub-Saharan Africa are outlined and then the World Food Programme (WFP), an organisation which is effectively working towards the achievement of this MDG, is introduced representatively for other organisations employing one or more of these strategies. In this paper the current food price crisis, climate change

---

[3]The GHI is a multidimensional approach of IFPRI to measuring hunger and malnutrition. The index ranks countries on a 100-point scale, with 0 being the best score (no hunger) and 100 being the worst. GHI currently lists 88 countries. All countries below a GHI of 5 are not included in the index.

and the presumably upcoming energy crisis are identified as three major threats to the extreme poverty and hunger MDG. Therefore, in the second section it is analysed in which way these threats affect or will probably affect the achievement of this goal.

4.1. Strategies and Actions

A research group around Haddad and Martorell (2002) from the *International Food Policy Research Institute* (IFPRI) identifies *'low-productivity agriculture where the poor live, lack of income, poor governance, conflict and war, human immunodeficiency virus/acquired immunodeficiency syndrome and natural disasters'* (3435) as the main causes of increasing poverty and hunger in sub-Saharan Africa. The authors stress that the hunger downward spiral in this region can only be decelerated when major changes will be conducted in the areas of investment, technology, and national-level institution and governance structures. Rosegrant and Meijer (2002) state that major investments have to be undertaken in the five key sectors irrigation, rural roads, agricultural research, clean water provision, and education. According to the authors' calculations annual investments in the amount of US$ 35 billion in these sectors will be necessary to achieve substantial food security improvements and to meet the poverty and hunger MDG. Thomson (2002) stresses the importance to invest in biotechnological research, particularly in crops that are drought tolerant, rich in micronutrients, and that are resistant to viruses, to both preharvest and postharvest fungi, and to insects. Rukuni (2002) investigated public policy trends across Africa and comes to the conclusion that *'African nations have to pursue policies and strategies that promote long-term growth while at the same time offering short-term safety nets for the poorest of the poor'* (3447). An appropriate strategy for growth and development would be to increase agricultural productivity in the smallholder commercial sector in order to simultaneously increase food availability and rural incomes and to lower the price of food for all net food purchasers in both rural and urban areas. However, Rukuni (2002) stresses that it is equally important for governments to adopt complementary food security policies that guarantee food security at the household level by increasing the probability of food access by the vulnerable groups.

Numerous organisations within the UN System, national governments, NGOs, and the private sector, who fight against poverty and hunger and thereby contributing to reach the poverty and hunger MDG include one or the other strategy as outlined above. Because a detailed description of all would go far beyond the scope of this paper, only one example is provided at this point. The WFP represents a good example, as it is the world's largest humanitarian organisation and by virtue of its commitment to the poverty and hunger MDG (WFP 2008). In 2007, WFP spent US$ 2.7 billion to run 35 country programmes, 19 development projects, 44 emergency operations, 69 relief and recovery operations, and 33 special operations, numbering 200 projects in total. Within these projects the organisation distributed 3.3 million metric tons (mt) of food to 86.1 million people in 80 countries. 15.3 million people were aided in emergency operations during conflicts and after natural disasters, especially in Sudan where WFP assisted up to 3 million beneficiaries in Darfur alone; in Uganda after catastrophic floods; or in the Sahel after being hit by drought and/or conflict. To strengthen developing country economies WFP spent US$ 612 million buying food in these regions, thereby providing income for farmers, and encouraging the development of local markets. To combat malnutrition of children and childhood mortality the organisation assisted 53.6 million children in WFP operations, in which 19.3 million children were provided with food rations within the scope of its school feeding programmes, and 5.7 million malnourished children received special nutritional support (WFP 2007b).

4.2. Major Threats

Even though numerous organisations and governments are currently working towards the achievement of the extreme poverty and hunger MDG and have produced certain successes, current economic and environmental developments are threatening this goal. Those threats identified as most urgent in this paper have all more or less to do with energy and petroleum in particular and have the potential to wreck the results already achieved. What follows is an analysis in which way these threats affect or will probably affect the achievement of the extreme poverty and hunger MDG.

4.2.1. Food Price Crisis

One major threat to achieve the extreme poverty and hunger MDG is the current worldwide food price crisis. In 2002 food prices were rising for the first time after decades of decline. Since then this trend continued, and from 2006 onwards food prices increased particularly steeply. In 2006 the Food and Agriculture Organisation (FAO) food price index[4] rose by 9% in

---

[4]The food price index consists of the average of the 6 commodity group price indices of meat, dairy, cereals, oils

2006, 24% in 2007, and even by 51% in 2008 (FAO 2009, Fig. 4.1.). The increase had affected virtually all food commodities, albeit to different degrees. With reference to 2003, in 2008 prices of wheat and poultry had doubled, prices of maize and butter had tripled, and the price of rice had even more than quadrupled (IFPRI 2008). The *High-Level Task Force (HLTF) on the Global Food Security Crisis* of the UN (2008b) states that the crisis is not the result of a specific climate shock or other emergency, but rather the *'cumulative effects of long-term trends and more recent factors, including supply and demand dynamics and responses which have caused further price increases and higher price volatility'* (1). Among these trends and factors HLTF (UN 2008b), IFPRI (2008) and the World Bank (2008a) identify harvest losses of

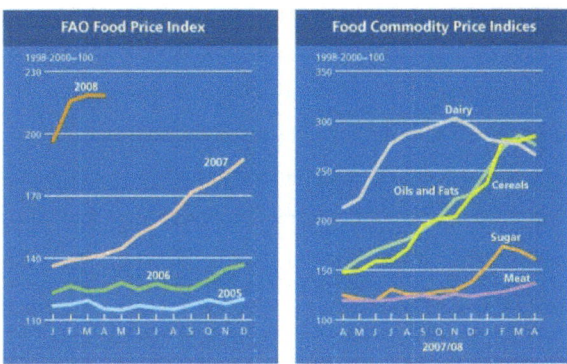

Figure 4.1. The FAO Price Index (Source: FAO 2008)

major grain producing countries due to extreme weather events, rising oil prices, declining private investments in agriculture, the conversion of farmland to non-agricultural uses due to urbanisation, increasing demand for biofuels, and speculation on stock markets as the leading causes of the crisis.

Those most affected by the current food price crisis are poor people in both urban and rural areas in developing countries. Many are net-buyers of food, who were estimated to spend up to three quarters of the incomes on staple food even before the crisis occurred (World Bank 2008b). Rising food prices are steadily increasing the proportion of their expenditure allocated to food, and thereby decreasing their ability to obtain other essential goods and services, such as health care and education. Many people who were comparatively better off before the crisis appeared are now being pushed below the poverty

---

and fats, and of sugar. These are weighted with the average export shares of each of the groups for 2002-2004 (FAO 2009).

line, as they are no longer able to pay the rising prices for food commodities. The UN (2008c) even estimates that an alarmingly high number of 100 million people are struck in that way, most of them living in sub-Saharan Africa and Southern Asia.

Since August 2008 the FAO notice a decline from the record levels of world prices of major agricultural commodities, some even by 50% from their recent peaks. As the prices have fallen farther and faster than could be explained through production gains alone, the organisation considers the financial crisis, the halving of world crude oil prices and the appreciation of the US dollar as the underlying causes responsible for the price slide (FAO 2008). However, despite the positive development in international food markets, domestic prices in developing countries remain generally very high and in some cases even reaching new records. According to FAO's (2009) latest analysis prices of rice are much higher than 12 months earlier in every African country south of the Sahara. Prices of maize, millet and sorghum are higher than they were 12 months earlier in about 89% of these countries, and wheat and wheat products are in 71% countries higher than 12 months before. Moreover, as the current decline of world food prices apparently reflects a slow-down in economic growth that constricts demand, FAO (2008) stresses that lower prices must be associated with more poverty and hunger rather than less.

4.2.2. Climate Change

Another major threat to the extreme poverty and hunger MDG pose the altering of the world's climate. In its *Fourth Assessment Report* the Intergovernmental Panel on Climate Change (IPCC 2007) defines climate change as *'a change in the state of the climate that can be identified by changes in the mean and/or the variability of its properties, and that persists for an extended period, typically decades or longer'* (30). Climate change refers predominantly to global warming and its effects on the environment. The IPCC (2007) report states that in the period between 1995 and 2006, 11 years rank among the 12 warmest years since the beginning of recording of the global surface temperature in 1850. Even though the authors of the IPCC report admit that the current climatic development may also be induced partly by natural variability it identifies human activities as the main driver of climate change. In this connection global emissions of long-lived greenhouse gases (GHGs) are the primary causes of global warming with carbon dioxide (CO_2) as the most important anthropogenic GHG, as it represents 77% of total GHG emissions. Between 1970 and 2004 its annual emissions have grown from 21 to 38 gigatonnes, which is an increase by about 80%. As a result of the rapid increase in CO_2 emission, concentrations of this GHG in the atmosphere increased from approximately 280 parts per million (ppm) in pre-industrial times to 382 ppm in 2006 (EPA 2009, Fig 4.2.). According to the IPCC report, in the long run the world will face an increase in global average warming attributed to GHG emissions in the range of 2 to 4.5°C, with a best estimate of approximately 3°C.

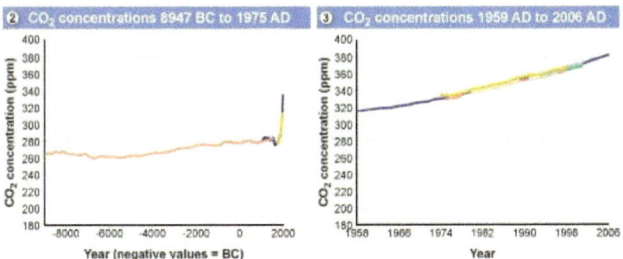

Figure 4.2. Atmospheric concentrations of CO_2 in pre-industrial times and in recent years (Source: EPA 2009).

Impacts of this drastic increase in temperature are manifold and are observable already today at all continents and most oceans: The global average sea level rises due to the melting of glaciers and ice sheets in both polar regions and Greenland, precipitation over most mid- and high-latitudes of the northern hemisphere increased, as well as the intensity and frequency of droughts, floods and severe storms.

To Africa the current development poses a great threat as it is probably the most vulnerable continent to climate change and climate variability. Boko et al. (2007), who are members of the Working Group II of the IPCC, enumerate in their contribution to the *Fourth Assessment Report* endemic poverty, limited access to capital, markets, infrastructure, and technology, ecosystem degradation, and complex disasters and conflicts as the main reasons why Africa's major economic sectors are vulnerable to current climate sensitivity. As for these reasons Africa has little adaptive and coping capacities, it is highly likely that climate change will have negative impacts on its societies and environments. Boko et al. (2007) stress that the ongoing increase in temperature will make agriculture even more challenging in those African countries already facing semi-arid conditions, as climate change will be likely to reduce the length of growing season and will force large regions of marginal agriculture out of production. In some countries this could result in yield reductions by as much as 50% already in 2020. In addition, it is likely that climate change will aggravate the water stress currently faced by some countries, so that the limits of their economically usable land-based water resources will be exceeded by several more African countries in the same year. Moreover, Boko et al. (2007) emphasise that sea-level rise could result in low-lying lands being inundated, particularly the coasts of eastern Africa, which will probably increase the high socio-economic as well as the physical vulnerability of coastal cities. Flooding will also facilitate the expansion of malaria and other water-borne diseases. There is evidence as well, that changes in temperature and precipitation in the East African highlands and southern Africa could alter the geographical distribution of malaria, making previously unsuitable areas suitable for malaria. Altogether, it seems obvious that if no solutions to these problems can be found it is likely that in sub-Saharan Africa poverty, hunger, and disease will increase in the future.

4.3. Energy Crisis

Another major threat to the extreme hunger and poverty MDG is the upcoming production peak of crude oil, in science literature commonly known as *Peak Oil*. When in 1956 geophysicist Marion King Hubbert (1956) warned the United States that the production peak of crude oil would occur within the country between 1966 and 1972, most economists, oil companies, and government agencies dismissed his prediction – particularly against the background that the United States was by then the biggest producer of crude oil in the world

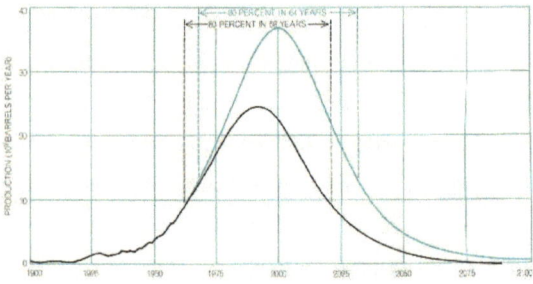

Figure 4.3. Hubbert's Peak (Source: Hubbert 1971: 39)

and did not face any difficulties in increasing its production (Tsoskounoglou et al. 2008). But his critics became silent when in 1970 the peak was actually reached, and from then on production steadily declined. Following his prediction of the US production peak, in 1971, on the basis of available data on total recoverable world petroleum reserves, Hubbert (1971) forecasted that the world production of crude oil would peak around 2000 (Fig. 4.3.). That he

28

was wrong this time was because in his model he did not incorporate the artificial limitations to oil production due to political constraints imposed by OPEC in 1973 and 1980 (Almeida et al. 2009). Having more accurate data at hand, in 1998, geologist Colin J. Campbell and oil engineer Jean Laherrère – Hubbert's most prominent followers – predicted in their influential paper *The End of Cheap Oil* that the world production of crude oil *'will peak during the first decade of the 21st century'* (Campbell and Laherrère 1998: 81). This prediction is accepted by many analysts today, as most of their own forecasts are focused around 2010 (Almeida et al. 2009)

These predictions are not mere assertions of prophets, but rely on careful analyses of leading oil geologists, geophysicists and petroleum industry experts. Their analyses are mainly based upon the Peak Oil theory originally introduced by Hubbert. The Hubbert peak theory, as it is usually called, holds that for any given geographical area, including the planet as a whole, the production of crude oil grows, reaches a maximum, and then gradually declines to zero. Fossil fuel production therefore follows a bell-shaped curve (Hubbert 1956 and 1971). The maximum of crude oil production is reached when about 50% of the ultimate production volume has been extracted. For the whole world this will be the case when about half of all Ultimately Recoverable Resources (URR) have been exploited. Given the fact that new discoveries of oilfields have been declining for many years, which therefore allow assessments with comparative accuracy, most analysts estimate the URR to be in the region of 2-3 trillion barrels. As we have exploited roughly 1 trillion barrels until today and are currently consuming 30 billion barrels a year, the Peak is assumed to be less than 15 years away (Tsoskounoglou et al. 2008). The German branch of Campbell's and Laherrère's *Association for the Study of Peak Oil and Gas* (ASPO) even suggests that Peak Oil did already occur in 2005 (ASPO Deutschland 2007).

Almost every aspect of the world's societies is heavily dependent on oil, since it is the leading source of energy in the world's transportation system. Moreover, it is used to generate electricity, to provide power for industry and agriculture, and as a feedstock for the manufacture of other materials, such as lubricants, plastics, artificial fibres and fertilisers (Hanlon and McCartney 2008, Klare 2001). As the world's population is increasing dramatically and because of the rapid industrialisation in the developing areas of Asia and Latin America demand for oil is rising steadily, currently at more than 2% a year. When the Peak is reached, it is estimated that production from existing oil wells will decline at an

29

average rate of 4-6% (Tsoskounoglou et al. 2008). It is apparent from this numbers that at this point supply of crude oil will by no means be able to keep up with demand. As a consequence, oil prices will rise significantly, reducing the feasibility of international trade for goods and services. This entails that Peak Oil will not only lead to a global economic depression of unprecedented dimension, but it will also lead to increased political tensions and conflicts, as availability of crude oil diminishes (Hanlon and McCartney 2008, Klare 2001). The combined effects of global recession and war due to decreasing energy supply will almost inevitable increase the proportion of people living in absolute poverty in the developing countries. For this reason, the *High-Level Task Force on UK Energy, Climate Change and Development Assistance* (2007) recently warned that the energy crisis following Peak Oil has the potential to wipe out MDG progress.

5. Conclusions

As it was demonstrated in this paper famines are caused due to a combination of several failures within a food system. The trigger must not necessarily be a natural disaster, but it can also be a socio-political event triggering a famine. This was confirmed by employing the Panarchy framework, a system theory recently introduced by Gunderson and Holling (2002). It was shown that the theory is useful not only to explain famine causation, but also the fact that not every calamity is triggering a famine, when appropriate counteractions are initiated by higher levels of the food system. When these actions fail or when no solutions are at hand the whole food system may collapse. The result is then an emerging famine. However, the examples of Kenya and Ethiopia have shown that several difficulties arise when one attempts to implement the Panarchy framework. This is due to certain weaknesses of the theory, especially those trying to impose concepts originally introduced in the natural sciences onto the social sciences. Nevertheless, the Panarchy framework proved to be useful when holistically regarded, and for this reason it is worthwhile to further elaborate this theory. Yet, although some authors successfully employed Panarchy in the context of famine causation, at this stage of development its validity cannot be fully confirmed.

When a food system collapses and famine emerges, mortality increases due to severe malnutrition and hunger-related diseases. As it was indicated in this paper the majority of the famine victims are dying from infectious diseases, as the immune system of malnourished persons becomes weakened which results in increased susceptibility to potentially fatal diseases. While the starvation model fully accepts the relationship between destitution, malnutrition and mortality, the health crisis model runs contrary to it and rejects that excess mortality is the direct outcome of destitution. Instead, it suggests that famine causes death in parallel to destitution, as an increased exposure to infectious diseases exists. However, the popular view of the starvation model was used in this paper, as the health crisis model is highly debatable – although its validity cannot be rejected.

Sub-Saharan Africa is the only region in the world where poverty and hunger is increasing. If the structural problems this continent faces cannot be resolved it is unlikely that it will meet the extreme poverty and hunger MDG. Nevertheless, UN Secretary General Ban Ki-moon recently declared: 'Looking ahead to 2015 and beyond, there is no question that we can achieve the overarching goal: we can put an end to poverty' (Ban Ki-moon in UN 2008a). It is true that millions of people could be raised out of poverty since the Millennium Declaration was resolved. But these successes were achieved due mainly to economic improvements in Asia. On the African continent poverty, hunger and disease still remain a sad reality. Moreover, the world's current challenges, such as the worldwide food price crisis, global climate change and the presumably upcoming energy crisis further threaten this goal in Africa. In this respect, the statement of the Secretary General appears to be rather overconfident.

6. Bibliography

ABEL, Nick, David H. M. Cumming & John M. Anderies. *Collapse and Reorganization in Social-Ecological Systems: Questions, Some Ideas, and Policy Implications.* Ecology and Society 11 (1): 17. [online] URL: http://www.ecologyandsociety.org/vol11/iss1/art17/ [01.04.2009].

ALMEIDA, Pedro de & Pedro D. Silva. *The Peak of Oil Production – Timings and Market Recognition.* Energy Policy 37, 1267-1276 (2009).

Ambrus, Julian L., Sr. & Julian L. Ambrus, Jr. *Nutrition and Infectious Diseases in Developing Countries and Problems of Acquired Immunodeficiency Syndrome.* Exp Biol Med 229: 464-472 (2004).

ASPO Deutschland. *Peak Oil is now!* 2007. [online] URL: http://www.aspo-germany.org/ [08.05.2009]

BADKHEN, Anna. *Famine in East Africa. Littlest Victims of Drought, Poverty.* In: The San Francisco Chronicle, 30.03.2006, A -1. [online] URL: http://www.sfgate.com/cgi-bin/article.cgi?file=/c/a/2006/03/30/MNGLEI0INB1.DTL [12.05.2009]

BERKES, Fikret & Carl Folke. *Back to the Future: Ecosystem Dynamics and Local Knowledge.* In: Lance Gunderson, C. Holling (Eds.). *Panarchy: Understanding Transformations in Human and Natural Systems.* Island Press, Washington, DC: 2002.

BERKLEY, James et al. *Assessment of Severe Malnutrition Among Hospitalized Children in Rural Kenya: Comparison of Weight for Height and Mid Upper Arm Circumference.* JAMA 294: 5, 591-597 (2005).

Boko, M. et al. *Africa. Climate Change 2007: Impacts, Adaptation and Vulnerability. Contribution of Working Group II to the Fourth Assessment Report of the Intergovernmental Panel on Climate Change*, M.L. Parry et al. (Eds.), Cambridge University Press, Cambridge, 433-467 (2007).

BRAUN, Joachim von, Tesfaye Teklu & Patrick Webb. *Famine in Africa. Causes, Responses, and Prevention.* The John Hopkins University Press, Baltimore and London: 1999

CAMPBELL, Colin J. & Jean H. Laherrère. *The End of Cheap Oil.* Scientific American, 78-83 (1998)

CARPENTER, Steve et al. *From Metaphor to Measurement: Resilience of What to What?* Ecosystems 4: 8, 765-781 (2001).

CDCP. *Famine-affected, refugee, and displaced populations: Recommendations for public health issues.* MMWR Recomm Rep 41: 1-76 (1992). [online] URL: http://www.cdc.gov/mmwr/preview/mmwrhtml/00019261.htm [20.04.2009].

COMENETZ, Joshua & César Caviedes. *Climate variability, political crises, and historical population displacements in Ethiopia.* Environment Hazards 4, 113-127 (2002).

DE ONIS, Mercedes & Monika Blössner. *The World Health Organization Global Database on Child Growth and Malnutrition: methodology and applications.* International Journal of Epidemiology 32, 518-526 (2003).

DE WAAL, Alex. *Famine that Kills. Darfur, Sudan.* Revised Edition. Oxford University, New York: 2005 [1989].

DEVEREUX, Stephen. *Famine in the Twentieth Century.* IDS Working Paper 105: 2000.

DYSON, Tim & Cormac ó Gráda. *Famine Demography. Perspectives from the Past and Present.* Oxford University Press, New York: 2002

EKWEAGWU, E., A. E. Akwu & E. Madukwe. *The role of micronutrients in child health: A review of the literature.* African Journal of Biotechnology 7: 21, 3804-3810 (2008).

ERICKSEN, Polly J. *What Is the Vulnerability of a Food System to Global Environmental*

Change? Ecology and Society 13 (2): 14 (2008).
[online] URL: http://www.ecologyandsociety.org/vol13/iss2/art14/ [26.02.2009]
EPA. *Atmospheric Concentrations of Greenhouse Gases in Geological Time and in Recent Years*. 2009.
[online] URL: http://www.epa.gov/climatechange/science/recentac_majorghg.html#fig1 [19.05.2009]
FAO. *Food Outlook. Global Market Analysis*. Global Information and Early Warning System on Food and Agriculture. 2008 (2).
------. *New FAO database confirms that domestic prices in developing countries remain very high*. In: *Crop Prospects and Food Situation*. FAO Report 2, April 2009
[online] URL: http://www.fao.org/docrep/011/ai481e/ai481e05b.htm [29.04.2009]
FOLKE, Carl et al. *Resilience and Sustainable Development: Building Adaptive Capacity in a World of Transformations*. Scientific Background Paper on Resilience for the process of The World Summit on Sustainable Development on behalf of The Environmental Advisory Council to the Swedish Government: 2002.
FRASER, Evan D. G. *Social Vulnerability and Ecological Fragility: Building Bridges between Social and Natural Sciences Using the Irish Potato Famine as a Case Study*. Conservation Ecology 7 (2): 9 (2003). [online] URL: http://www.consecol.org/vol7/iss2/art9 [02.03.2009]
FRASER, Evan D. G. *Travelling in antique lands: using past famines to develop an adaptability/resilience framework to identify food systems vulnerable to climate change*. Climatic Change 83, 495-514 (2007)
FRASER, Evan D. G., Warren Mabee & Frank Figge. *A framework for assessing the vulnerability of food systems to future shocks*. Futures 37, 465-479 (2005)
GUNDERSON, Lance. & Crawford S. Holling. *Resilience and Adaptive Cycles*. In: Lance Gunderson, C. Holling (Eds.). *Panarchy: Understanding Transformations in Human and Natural Systems*. Island Press, Washington, DC: 2002.
GUNDERSON, Lance, Crawford S. Holling & Garry D. Peterson. *Sustainability and Panarchies*. In: Lance Gunderson, C. Holling (Eds.). *Panarchy: Understanding Transformations in Human and Natural Systems*. Island Press, Washington, DC: 2002.
HADDAD, Lawrence & Reynaldo Martorell. *Feeding the World in the Coming Decades Requires Improvements in Investment, Technology and Institutions*. Symposium: Feeding the World in the Coming Decades. In: The American Society for Nutritional Sciences 132, 3435-3436 (2002)
HANLON, P. & G. McCartney. *Peak Oil: Will it be public health's greatest challenge?* In: Public Health 122, 647-652 (2008).
HLTF on UK Energy Security, Climate Change and Development Assistance. *Energy, Politics, and Poverty. A Strategy for Energy Security, Climate Change and Development Assistance*. Oxford University: 2007.
HOLLING, Crawford S. *Understanding the Complexity Economic, Ecological, and Social Systems*. Ecosystems 4: 5, 390-405 (2001).
------. *Resilience and stability of ecological systems*. Annual Review of Ecology and Systematics 4, 1-23 (1973).
HUBBERT, Marion King. *Nuclear Energy and the Fossil Fuels*. Shell Development Company. Exploration and Production Research Division. Publication No. 95. Houston, Texas: 1956.
------. *The Energy Resources of the Earth*. In: Energy and Power, a Scientific American Book. W. H. Freeman & Co., San Francisco, 31–40: 1971. [online]
URL: http://www.hubbertpeak.com/Hubbert/energypower/ [08.05.2009]
IFPRI. *Global Hunger Index: The Challenge of Hunger 2008*. Klaus von Grebmer et al. (Ed.).

Bonn, Washington D.C., Dublin: 2008

IPCC. *Fourth Assessment Report of the Intergovernmental Panel on Climate Change*. Synthesis Report. M.L. Parry et al. (Eds.), Cambridge University Press, Cambridge: 2007.

KASPERSON, Roger E. and Jeanne X. Kasperson. *Climate Change, Vulnerability and Social Justice*. Risk and Vulnerability Programme, Stockholm Environment Institute: 2001.

KLARE, Michael T. *Resource Wars. The New Landscape of Global Conflict*. Owl Books, New York: 2001

KOPPEL, Johan van de et al. *Catastrophic vegetation shifts and soil degradation in terrestrial grazing systems*. TREE 12: 9, 352-356 (1997).

LANG, Mark. *Ethiopian food crisis: a family's struggle*. In: Times Online, 30.07.2008. [online] URL: http://www.timesonline.co.uk/tol/comment/faith/article4428094.ece [12.05.2009]

MÜLLER, Olaf & Michael Krawinkel. *Malnutrition and health in developing countries*. CMAJ 173: 3, 279-286 (2005).

NOWAK, Rachel. *African droughts "triggered by western pollution"*. New Scientist (online edition) (2002).

NYAMWANGE, Monica. *Famine Mitigation in Kenya: Some Practices, Impact and Lessons*. Middle States Geographer 28, 37-44 (1995).

OBRIST, B, Iteba N, Lengeler C, Makemba A, Mshana C, et al. *Access to Health Care in Contexts of Livelihood Insecurity: A Framework for Analysis and Action*. PLoS Med 4:1, 1584-1588 (2007): e308. doi:10.1371/journal.pmed.0040308.

OSTROM, Elinor. Review article to: Lance Gunderson, Crawford S. Holling & Garry D. Peterson. *Panarchy: Understanding Transformations in Human and Natural Systems*. Island Press, Washington, DC: 2002. In: Ecological Economics 9, 488-491 (2004).

ROSEGRANT, Mark W. & Siet Meijer. *Appropriate Food Policies and Investments could reduce child malnutrition by 43 % in 2020*. Symposium: Feeding the World in the Coming Decades. In: The American Society for Nutritional Sciences 132, 3437-3440 (2002).

SALAMA, Peter et al. *Malnutrition, Measles, Mortality, and the Humanitarian Response During a Famine in Ethiopia*. JAMA 286: 5, 563-571 (2001).

SCHAIBLE, Ulrich E. & Stefan H. E. *Kaufmann. Malnutrition and Infection: Complex Mechanisms and Global Impacts*. PLoS Med 4(5): e115. doi:10.1371/journal.pmed.0040115 (2007)

SCHEFFER, Marten et al. *Catastrophic shifts in ecosystems*. Review Paper. Nature 413, 591-596 (2001).

SEAL, Andrew & Claudine Prudhon. *Assessing micronutrient deficiencies in emergencies. Current practice and future directions*. Nutrition Information in Crisis Situations. United Nations System Standing Committee on Nutrition, 2007.

SHANKAR, Anuraj H. *Nutritional Modulation of Malaria Morbidity and Mortality*. The Journal of Infectious Diseases 182 (Suppl 1), 37-53 (2000).

SPERANZA, Chinwe I., Boniface Kiteme & Urs Wiesmann. *Droughts and famines: The underlying factors and the causal links among agro-pastoral households in semi-arid Makueni district, Kenya*. Global Environmental Change 18, 220-233 (2008).

SPHERE PROJECT. *Humanitarian Charter and Minimum Standards in Disaster Response*. Steering Committee for Humanitarian Response. Geneva: 2004

SWINDALE, Anne & Paula Bilinsky. *Household Dietary Diversity Score (HDDS) for Measurement of Household Food Access: Indicator Guide*. Food and Nutrition Technical Assistance Project (FANTA). Academy for Educational Development. Washington, DC: 2005

RUKUNI, Mandivamba. *Africa: Addressing Growing Threats to Food Security*. Symposium:
Feeding the World in the Coming Decades. In: The American Society for Nutritional
Sciences 132, 3443-3448 (2002)

TSOSKOUNOGLOU, Miltos, George Ayerides, Efi Tritopoulou. *The Ende of Cheap Oil: Current
Status and Prospects*. In: Energy Policy 36, 3797-3806 (2008).

THOMSON, Jennifer A. *Research Need to Improve Agricultural Productivity and Food
Quality, with Emphasis on Biotechnology*. Symposium: *Feeding the World in the Coming
Decades*. In: The American Society for Nutritional Sciences 132, 3441-3442 (2002).

TURNER, B. L. et al. *A framework for vulnerability analysis in sustainability science*. PNAS 100:
14, 8074-8079 (2003).

UN. *United Nations Millennium Declaration*. Resolution adopted by the General Assembly,
55th session. 2000.

------. *Global Public Health and the Eradication of Poverty*. The Fourth Forum on the
Eradication of Poverty. United Nations Headquarters, New York: 2008a

------. *Comprehensive Framework for Action*. High-Level Task Force on the Global Food
Security Crisis. 2008b

------. *The Millennium Development Goals Report*. New York: 2008c

UNDP. *Kenya Natural Disaster Profile*. 2004.
[online] URL: http://www.ke.undp.org/KenyaDisasterProfile.pdf [29.03.2009]

UNICEF. *The State of the World's Children*. Oxford University Press, New York: 1998

UN Millennium Project. *Halving hunger: it can be done*. Summary version of the report of the
Task Force on Hunger. The Earth Institute at Columbia University, New York, USA (2005).

------. *Fast Facts: The Faces of Poverty*. 2006. [online]
URL: http://www.unmillenniumproject.org/documents/3-MP-PovertyFacts-E.pdf
[26.04.2009]

UNRUH, Jon D. *The Dilemma of African Agrobiodiversity: Ethiopia and the Role of Food
Insecurity Conservation*. United Nations University: 2001.
[online] URL: http://www.unu.edu/env/plec/cbd/montreal/papers/unruh.pdf [08.03.2009]

WALKER, Brian et al. *Exploring Resilience in Social-Ecological Systems Through Comparative
Studies and Theory Development: Introduction to the Special Issue*. Ecology and Society 11
(1): 12 (2006a). [online] URL: *http://www.ecologyandsociety.org/vol11/iss1/art12/*
[15.03.2009].

WALKER, Brian et al. *A Handful of Heuristics and Some Propositions for Understanding
Resilience in Social-Ecological Systems*. Ecology and Society 11 (1): 13 (2006b)
[online] URL: *http://www.ecologyandsociety.org/vol11/iss1/art13/* [01.04.2009].

WATERLOW, J. C. *Protein-energy malnutrition: the nature and extent of the problem*. Clinical
Nutrition 16 (Suppl 1), 3-9 (1997).

WEBB, Patrick & Andrew Thorne-Lyman. *Micronutrients in Emergencies*. Food Policy and
Applied Nutrition Programme. Discussion Paper No. 32. Tufts University Boston,
Massachusetts: 2005. [online]
URL: http://nutrition.tufts.edu/docs/pdf/fpan/wp32micronutrients_in_emergencies.pdf
[04.04.2009]

WFP. *World Hunger Series 2007: Hunger and Health*. Gutenberg Press, Malta: 2007a

------. 2007 in Review. Division of Communications and Public Policy Strategy. Rome
Italy: 2007b

------. *Strategic Plan 2008-2011*. Division of Communications and Public Policy Strategy. Rome
Italy: 2008

WHO. *Communicable diseases and severe food shortage situations.* World Health Organization Communicable Diseases Working Group on Emergencies (CD-WGE). 2005. [online] URL: http://www.who.int/malaria/docs/CDs_severe_food_shortages.pdf [17.04.2009]

------. *Nutrient requirements for people living with HIV/AIDS. Report of a technical consultation.* Geneva: 2003.

------. *The World Health Report 2002. Reducing Risk, Promoting Healthy Life.* Geneva: 2002.

------. *Management of the Child with a serious Infection or severe Malnutrition. Guidelines for Care at the first-referral Level in developing Countries.* Department of Child and Adolescent Health and Development. 2000.

------. *Physical Status: The Use and Interpretation of Anthropometry.* Report of WHO Expert Committee. WHO Technical Report Series 854. Geneva: 1995.

WOODRUFF, BA & A. Duffield. *Anthropometric assessment of nutritional status in adolescent populations in humanitarian emergencies.* European Journal of Clinical Nutrition 56: 1108-1118 (2002).

WORLD BANK. *A Note on Rising Food Prices.* Development Prospects Group: 2008a

------. *Implications of Higher Global Food Prices for Poverty in Low-Income Countries.* Development Research Group, Trade Team: 2008b

YOUNG, Oran R. et al. *The globalization of socio-ecological systems: An agenda for scientific research.* Global Environmental Change 16, 304-316 (2006).